CLARISA WASHOMA

Is Something Wrong with Me?

Because Silence Was Never Empty

First edition

This book was professionally typeset on Reedsy.
Find out more at reedsy.com

Contents

Preface

There was a time I asked myself daily... *Is something wrong with me?*

This book is more than my story, it's my testimony. It now serves as both a mirror and source of strength for anyone who has ever felt unseen and not enough.

I didn't write it because I had all the answers. I wrote it because I found peace in asking better questions.

Introduction

Written from a mother's heart.

This book is a long love letter. It's a guide. A time capsule. A bridge between generations. I wrote it for my daughter and other daughters out there.

Whether you're reading this today or 100 years from now, I hope you can feel my presence through every word. May these pages remind you that you were always seen, always worthy, and more than enough - even if life doesn't make sense right now, trust yourself that all things will work for the greater good.

This book is proof that transformation is possible. It's not a fairy-tale or theory, it's a lived experience. Through my own pain, questions, healing, and faith, I discovered the power of what was already within me.

To my daughter: you changed me in ways words will never fully explain. As I write this, you're just two years old. But your presence has already made me better. Don't ever lose sight of that.

To you, the reader: I hope we laugh together, cry together, and most of all - heal together. Because no matter what life throws your way, the journey to wholeness will always begin within.

I hope my story serves as a foundation and inspiration for you to connect from within. Although we are all on different journeys and experience life differently, one thing we will always have in common is our emotions and how they can nurture our thoughts to either liberate or destroy us.

So if you're ready, let's begin.

This is the moment you choose to *liberate yourself.*

Author's Note

This book is based on lived experiences and spiritual insights. While it contains personal reflections, the author is not a licensed therapist, counsellor, or minister. The intention is to offer healing through storytelling, not to replace professional guidance.

I

When Life Stops Making Sense

There comes a moment when everything you once knew starts to fall apart, slowly at first and then all at once. This part of my journey is about the unravelling: the pain that silenced me, the losses that broke me, and the survival that became my normal. I didn't choose this chapter, but I had to walk through it to find truth. This is where it all began.

1

The End of the Beginning

I wrote this book for the girl who walks into a room and doesn't know where she belongs.

I wrote this book for the one who sees beauty in everyone else - but not in herself.

I wrote this book for the one who dimmed her light so others could shine.

I wrote this book for the one who was never enough because she didn't show up like others.

I wrote this book for the one who absorbed pain like a sponge, silencing her voice - not out of weakness but because she understood pain...and it's power.

And finally, I wrote this book as a letter to the world, and to that one person - reminding them: ***Your freedom was always***

rooted in love. But it had to start with YOU.

Everything you have buried has always been the root of your strength.

The empty mirror wasn't there to shame you, it was waiting for you to stand in front of it and finally recognise: ***Everything you've been searching for has always been right in front of you.***

Give yourself Permission to be happy

It's amazing how much life can change if we stop living in our thoughts and start being present with ourselves. We spend so much time worrying about things that haven't happened yet and when the time arrives, it often doesn't unfold the way we imagined. By then, there's usually something new on our list that consumes us. When do we get to simply be human beings and exist in the now?

There is simple joy in waking up whole, feeling the sun on your face, holding your loved one's hand or sharing a meal - truly present, seeing love through their eyes of a heart that's still grounded of looking at love through the lens of a heart that's still and grounded. It draws us into a physiological state of LOVE, into a formless space - like the one who loved us before we were ever born.

If only you knew how much power and warmth you hold when you ground yourself!

2

The Day it All Started

When faith was quietly born.

I spent most of my life feeling like I was too ambitious.
Not because I thought I was better than anyone…
But because I couldn't stop dreaming.

There was always more I could see.
I wanted to build more.
I felt more was possible.

Yet here I was.
The "big moment" hadn't arrived.
No headline of success.
Just vision…and vibes.
(And did you catch that? The subtle negative thoughts slipping in)

Where do we begin?

May 2021

That's when it started to shift.

Not because something dramatic happened.

But because I finally… paused.

My parents said something simple that day: "Enjoy the process"

I remember it clearly.

I was in the garden with my parents at home.

And I wasn't having the success with my career the way I had planned.

I remember looking at my father asking;

"Why do I exist?"

I felt like a cloud.

Drifting.

Hopeless.

No direction.

And this part is hard to say but I'll say it anyway:

I never thought about taking my life.

But if someone had offered to end it for me…

I might have volunteered.

That's how far gone I felt.

And yet somehow…

That moment slowed me down.

I stopped listening to the world.

Started listening to the silence.

To the still, small voice inside.

Here is what I now know:

"Enjoy the process" isn't passive advice.
It's an invitation.
To breathe.
To reflect.
To trust that you're not behind.
And vision without pressure?
That's called faith.
And sometimes…
That's more than enough.

3

A Bike Ride and a Breakthrough

When joy found me in motion.

Of course, I didn't say any of that to my father at the time.
But he knew.
He saw it in the way I moved.
Or didn't.

He read between the silence.
Sometimes love says nothing and still hears everything.
That moment stayed with me.
Not for what he said but what it sparked inside me.

A question I couldn't shake:
What does it mean to enjoy the process?

I needed something to shift.
Something to get me out of my head and into my body.
So... I bought a bicycle.

If you know me, you know how wild that sounds.

That wasn't me.

But that was the point.

I remember calling a friend, just to hear the surprise in their voice.

"I'm going to give you a visit", they said.

That's when I knew… something was waking up.

The days that followed were different.

Not because life changed but because I did.

I started to feel something I hadn't felt in a long time:

JOY!

The wind on my face.

The music in my ears.

The movement.

No pressure. No finish line.

Just me, riding and dreaming.

For two months straight, I let myself exist in that space.

Somewhere between hope and healing.

And something magical happened…

I started to imagine again.

Recipes.

Textures.

Colours.

Ideas that felt doable.

Not distant.

Just me and my vision.

There was no loan.
No business plan.
No permission slip.
Just a girl in the kitchen, dreaming again.

As soon as Friday arrived.
I went to the supermarket with a different kind of excitement.
This wasn't just shopping.
This was a mission.
Each ingredient had a purpose.
I could already see the video before it existed.
Feeling the emotion behind each pour, each cut and sizzle.
When I got home, I set it all up:
Phone balanced above the spice cupboard.
LED light over the counter.
Pressed record.
Chopped my onions.
Staged every transition.
Poured myself into that plate.

When the meal was ready, I didn't eat for 30 minutes.
I just stared.
Did I really make that?

That was the birth of **Dine With Clarisa**.
Not just a page.
Not just a passion.
But a portal, back to myself.

And I realised something...

Joy doesn't have to be earned.
Sometimes it shows up when you finally stop performing.
When you just... play.

Finding yourself isn't always deep work.
Sometimes it's light work.
Whisking sauce. Dancing in socks.

Your soul knows what excites you.
Even when logic doesn't.

Stillness isn't failure.
It's space.
And sometimes, that space is sacred.

This was the beginning of something I didn't have language for yet.
But I knew it was good.
Because I was becoming.
Not just productive. Not just useful.

Alive.

4

The Quiet Exit of Confidence

When doubt walks in without knocking.

It started so well.
I was experimenting, editing, and recording.
Not to impress. Just for joy.

Each video felt like play.
I was learning. Growing.
Coming alive.

And then it happened.
One comment.
Just one.
Maybe they didn't mean it harshly.
But it landed.

And like a crack in a window.
The doubt slipped in.

"Maybe this isn't that good."
"Maybe I'm doing too much."
"Maybe I should stop"

And that's how it begins.

Confidence doesn't disappear all at once.
It fades.
Silently.
You hit a roadblock.
You hear something off.
You see someone else doing it "better".
And suddenly…
You forget why you started.

Becoming a master at dimming my own light, when expectations weren't met.
What if I dropped the expectations?
And…
What if joy was the goal… not perfection?

I started to recognise a pattern in my own emotions.
Expectations killed the spark.
But intention?
Intention kept it burning.

I allowed joy to be my measure.
And the process to be exactly that… enough.
Every time you show up with heart, you're winning.

Realisation:

I used to think confidence came from knowing.
Knowing what you're doing.
Knowing how it'll all turn out.

But I've learned…
Confidence comes from doing it anyway.
Even when you're unsure.
Even when the voice in your head starts whispering, "Who do you think you are?"

That version of me who began, full of hope and fire.
She wasn't naive.
She was brave.

And every time I choose to keep going,
I don't just build confidence.
I reclaim power.

5

The Pain of the Unspoken

Giving voice to what I once buried in silence.

Dine with Clarisa became my escape.

It gave me something to focus on - something to create, when I wasn't ready to confront the pain I had buried so deeply.

One sunny day in July 2021, I was trying to deepen my relationship with God.

A friend connected me to a kind woman, a Jehovah's Witness - with a voice so soft, so warm, it almost felt out of place in the storm I was living in.

We did a Bible study that day. I remember the verse: "Your word is a lamp for my feet, a light on my path" - *Psalms 119: 105*

We spoke about how we may not see the whole path, we're given enough light to always take the next step with faith that the Lord shall always go before us.

Sometimes it's not clarity we need, it's courage. One small step in the dark can change everything.

Her voice was peaceful but inside me, something was restless.

I remember thinking, last time I trusted God - he let me down.

One of the deepest wounds I've carried is the death of my mother.

We didn't get to spend much time together in person.

I was just a child, always writing her letters with hope.

At the end of every note, I'd write; " May God protect you until we meet again. Love Clarisa."

But that day never came.

Just months before I turned 18, a police officer finally delivered the news to one of my uncles.

After 2 weeks of searching for her, she was gone.

No goodbye. Just absence.

Why me?

That unanswered question lingered like a shadow, I couldn't outrun it.

The world had moved on.

Except me.

Sometimes grief has no closure. It just learns to live beside you.

Equally, grief isn't always loud. Sometimes it hides behind drive, performance, or even a smile.

But buried pain doesn't disappear - it just waits.

Since then I told myself I'd never love that deeply again. If I disappointed myself first, no one else could.

After the Bible study that day, I felt heavy. But I didn't want to sit in it.

It had been 11 years - I told myself I should be "over" it by now.

So I did what I knew how to do: I cooked.

I went to the supermarket, bought ingredients and on the shelf near the checkout was a vodka cocktail kit, on offer.

Perfect timing!

That day was different. I played one song on repeat, dancing in the kitchen while pain disguised as fun.

That bottle of vodka disappeared like water.

And what came next... was verbal fire.

Words I didn't plan to say. Emotions I didn't know I was still carrying.

They came sideways - aimed at the wrong person.

Unprocessed pain always finds an outlet. If you don't speak it, you will leak it.

And the longer you suppress it, the more violent it's exit becomes.

I don't remember what I said, but the next day the feedback made me realise: the resentment I carried in my heart was deep.

And yet my mind whispered, *"Oh well. We move"*

But God had started something that day.

Not just light on my path but light on my heart.

He was slowing me down, showing me that the burden I carried wasn't even mine.

Healing doesn't always look holy. Sometimes it looks like breaking down in the kitchen with a bottle in your hand.

But even then, grace still finds you.

It took me years to understand that being kind to yourself is the beginning of acceptance, of the things you cannot change and real healing.

Not avoiding the truth. Not numbing it. But letting it rise, and meeting it with compassion.

Forgiveness is not forgetting what happened.

It's remembering without reliving. It's choosing to be free.

6

When Grief Becomes a Shadow

Unprocessed pain shapes the way we love, trust, and show up.

Grief doesn't just break your heart.
It changes your blueprint.

When my mother died, something in me quietly folded in on itself.

I didn't just lose her, I lost a piece of safety I didn't even know I was depending on.

And without realising it, I started building my life around that hole.

No one noticed. Not even me.

Sometimes the pain we avoid becomes the foundation we build on. And then we wonder why nothing feels steady.

I didn't stop loving.
I just became more calculated about it.
I gave, but stayed alert.

I smiled, but scanned the room for signs of withdrawal.

I laughed, but also built walls, tall enough to keep disappointment out, yet just low enough for people to think they were in.

Grief taught me how to protect myself.

But it also tricked me into thinking that protection was peace.

Avoidance doesn't heal grief, it delays it.

And eventually, delayed grief finds a disguise: hyper-independence, overthinking, people-pleasing... silence.

There were moments in my adult life were I felt fully present - fully loved.

But then, something would shift.

A distance. A silence. An unmet expectation.

And suddenly I'd retreat - not physically, but emotionally.

As if I was rehearsing for another loss before it ever happened.

That's what grief does when it's unspoken.

It doesn't need permission to stay. It quietly camps in your habits, your triggers, your trust.

And here's the thing - I wasn't bitter.

I was just scared to believe in forever again.

Even the word "forever" felt fragile.

You start to wonder if joy is just a setup. If connection is a countdown.

And love? Love becomes the biggest risk of all.

Here's what I've started to learn and it took me years to get here:

Grief doesn't leave
But it can evolve.
It can move from a shadow to a memory.
From a wound to wisdom.
I'm not trying to "get over" my mother's death anymore.
I'm learning how to carry her differently.
Not as a question mark. But as a quiet strength.

7

The Day I Almost Said No

A love letter to the beginning you never saw, but came from.

To my daughter,

When I met your father, I was in the midst of finding myself.

Not in a dramatic, soul searching kind of way - more like the quiet type.

The kind of self-discovery where you're learning to speak to yourself gently.

You don't need every part of your life to make sense before you smile.

I didn't know I was ready for love.

And maybe I wasn't.

But that's the thing about love - sometimes, it arrives before the mirror reflects back someone you fully recognise.

That day my cousin (your aunt) insisted that I go to this music festival.

I had no energy for it but she wouldn't take no for an answer.

I remember everything that afternoon.

The outfit - a fitted jumpsuit, lashes on and make up done.

I looked good but if I'm honest... *I didn't feel it.*

My confidence was somewhere between "just show up" and "hold it together".

I wasn't in the mood to celebrate anything.

It was one of those moments where you feel like performing joy you haven't earned.

But I went.

And that's how the magic happens sometimes

You leave the house thinking you're just trying to get through the night... and the next chapter of life is waiting at the exit gate.

We were walking toward the car, laughing, winding down, when I saw him - your father.

He was just standing there. Quiet. Still.

Eyes locked on me. Saying nothing.

And in that moment, I don't know what came over me.

Maybe it was the part of me that had forgotten how to flirt.

Maybe it was the version of me that just wanted to feel free for a second.

But I walked right over, linked arms with him like we'd known each other for years and said

"Are you going to say something?"

We both laughed. It wasn't awkward. It was instant

The kind of laughter that feels like deja vu.

He walked me to the car. Asked for my number.

He wasn't my usual type, but something inside me didn't hesitate.

Something in me said yes before I had time to talk myself out of it.

And days passed.

Then weeks.

We spoke on the phone for hours.

Hung out, no pressure.

No pretending.

No needing to be the most "put together" version of myself.

He liked me when I was still unsure if I like me.

That meant something!

I didn't have to wear my "stage face".

Didn't have to dazzle.

Didn't have to perform softness or confidence or composure.

And for a woman - that's rare.

To be seen in the in-between.

To be loved in the becoming.

Not because you look like a magazine cover - but because something about you feels like home.

We fell in love the way morning turns into day

Not all at once, but unmistakably.

Quiet. Warm. Honest.

What a gift it was… to be wanted for my essence, not my image.
To be chosen when I wasn't auditioning.

That's where you came from,
Not a perfect story.
But a real one.
A soft, surprising love that began on a day I almost said no.

I hope one day when you read this, you always remember.
You were made in presence
Two people who met in transition, chose each other in truth,
and created something unforgettable - **you.**

II

The Awakening

Something within me began to stir, a quiet voice reminding me there was more. Becoming a mother cracked me open in ways I couldn't have prepared for. With it came an identity shift, a rebirth through baptism, and an invitation to do deeper inner work. This wasn't just the start of healing, it was the start of seeing myself clearly for the first time.

8

The Season of Grace

A quiet fairy-tale where love introduced me to myself.

Once upon a time, I became a carrier of my greatest blessing in April 2022.

Not just a child.

But stillness

Clarity

And the kind of love that doesn't knock, just moves in and rearranges everything.

Pregnancy was one of the most exciting chapters in my life. I had always wanted a child, so her timing came as no surprise.

It was a quiet, intentional yes to a new chapter of life.

But when the moment arrived, it demanded a different version of me.

One I had never met before.

I remember after my first appointment with my midwife, I took the "*do not stress*" very literally and it was the one time in my life were being in control was not an option because it was dependent on this miracle.

Stress had no invitation.

Negativity had no seat at the table.

And for the first time in my life, protecting someone else meant truly protecting myself.

Love had taken a physical form and it was growing inside of me.

What a beautiful and terrifying miracle.

I didn't know how much I needed her until my body became a home.

Each day wasn't perfect but it was intentional.

Every moment was guided by a silent promise:

"Whatever I didn't give myself... I will give to you."

But here's the truth that no one talks about:

As soon as I gave birth to my daughter, everything I had shelved for nine months - the fear, the pain, the pressure. It came back and sat me down.

Like old friends I didn't invite, ready to catch-up.

It's wild how life makes space for peace and then just as quickly, reminds you of everything you tried to forget.

Still I wouldn't trade that season for anything.

Because in that quiet fairy-tale.

I became the woman I was always meant to be.

Not perfect.
Not healed.
But I'm awake.

And maybe that's what grace really is:

A gentle, golden interruption that shows up in the middle of your becoming and whispers - "You're doing better than you think."

9

When Motherhood Unravels You

Motherhood shook something loose and I didn't know who I was anymore.

No one really talks about this part of becoming a mother.

Not the labour. Not the feeding schedules or sleep deprivation.

But the identity shift.

The slow, quiet unravelling of who you used to be,
while the world expects you to feel whole.

After my daughter was born, the love was overwhelming...but so was everything else.

The softness of her skin. The way she held my finger. The silent bond we shared.

But underneath that beauty was chaos I didn't know how to name.

I didn't lose myself in motherhood, I just couldn't find where

I'd gone.

There were moments of joy, of course.

But joy can still carry weight.

And mine did.

Because as my body healed, something inside of me felt misaligned.

I was excited, but also numb.

Present, but also far away.

I'd look in the mirror and wonder:

Is this me now?

Do I like her?

Can I still be who I was... or is she gone forever?

There were no breakdowns.

Just a quiet disorientation

I wasn't sad. But I wasn't rooted either.

It felt like I had been removed from the centre of my own life and placed at the edge, watching.

Observing.

Questioning.

If I'm no longer just Clarisa, now I'm a fiance and a mommy too - where do the three meet?

Motherhood gave me purpose.

But it also exposed parts of me I didn't know were still fragile.

The old me was used to striving, performing and pushing.

She knew how to chase things.

But the new me was being called to soften, to receive... to let things unfold.

And that felt terrifying.

I kept asking myself questions in the stillness.

Why do I miss who I was, even though she wasn't at peace?

Why do I feel guilty for not being grateful enough when I already have everything I prayed for?

What version of me is safe enough to show up now?

No one had answers for this.

Only the slow realisation that I had to figure this out on my own.

This wasn't depression or burnout.

It was *becoming* but in slow motion.

An identity suspended between different worlds.

And maybe that's what no one prepares you for:

That the most sacred transformations come without fanfare.

That motherhood doesn't just change your schedule - ***it changes your soul.***

10

The Baptism

Obedience before understanding.

December 2023.

It wasn't a dramatic moment.

There was no booming voice from heaven. No thunder in the clouds.

Just an invitation and a quiet yes.

My aunt encouraged me to get baptised while I was in Zimbabwe.

The pastor was visiting the city and it felt like the "right" thing to do.

I wasn't in a particularly spiritual place, since my last attempt.

My faith was present, but faint.

I said yes, not because I expected anything to happen but because... why not?

What's the worst that could happen?

At best my hair would get wet.

At worst I'd come home unchanged.

But God doesn't wait for us to understand.

He moves when we obey.

And obedience is often the loudest faith you can express when your heart feels quiet.

I remember standing in the water - neutral. Not emotional. Not expectant.

And yet… something was shifting.

January 2024 came

And without warning, everything around me began to move.

Not dramatically but deliberately.

The relationship with my partner grew tense.

The silence between us felt louder than any argument ever could.

And slowly, without realising I began the process of detachment not out of resentment but out of truth.

I could no longer carry the weight of keeping peace in places that felt like war.

Life changing moments often don't ask for permission. They just start removing what's not aligned.

And yet, the external world stayed the same.

Same house. Same job. Same smile.

But something invisible had awakened.

I wasn't reacting the same, I wasn't shrinking like before

I had questions I couldn't un-ask.

I remember looking at my daughter not just with love but with a heightened level of accountability.

How can I teach her who she is... if I don't even know who I am?

A sense of self that wouldn't let me go back to who I was.

I began to realise that growth isn't always a build-up, it's often a breakdown done quietly.

And the more I surrendered to what is, the more space I created for what could be.

I found myself going to the gym again. Not for appearance but for discipline.

I returned to work with a new kind of openness.

Started conversations I never would've before.

Volunteered. Listened. Spoke up.

I was different.

It didn't make sense at the time.

But something deeper was being reordered.

And all I could think, months later - while scrolling through my phone and stumbling across the baptism photo, was:

That was the moment my awakening accelerated.

I didn't feel it at the time.

But God wasn't looking for feeling.

He was watching for surrender.

And in the silence of that act, He moved.

Sometimes the moment you don't expect to matter becomes the hinge for your next season.

It wasn't my knowledge that activated the shift.

It was my obedience in not knowing.

And that's how grace moves - quietly.

Not always miraculous.

But in the ordinary moments when you say yes without a blueprint.

11

Identity Crisis

When the old you is gone - but the new you hasn't arrived.

If someone asked you, "Who are you?" - what would your response be?

I know that's a fully loaded question. But really think about it.
Most people respond with their relationship status, job role, their role in the world. But what if none of those apply anymore?
What if everything that once defined you... no longer does?

That was me.

A phone call to my second mother filled with silence.
She understood me without many words.
I remember that day because it was love that I didn't know I needed.
It was a language understood only by the heart.
"**Come back home**," she said.

May 2024

Back in my childhood home.

Single mother.

No idea what's coming next.

No plan to fall back on - just presence.

I felt like I was grieving someone I used to be but really didn't know how to mourn.

All I could think was: How did I get here? and more importantly...*who am I now?*

We were all a representation of love before life made us question it.

But the truth is, life was always designed that way.

Because how could we truly appreciate love if we had never known the opposite?

Maybe identity is meant to fall apart.

Maybe it's in rebuilding, we discover what's real.

Mine was falling apart in real time.

The titles blurred.

Clarisa.

Mom.

Daughter.

Fiance' - past tense.

And yet, in the stillness of all that loss, I noticed something I didn't expect:

Support.
Not perfect. But presence.

There was food on the table
Laughter in the hallway .
Someone to hold my daughter when I needed a moment to breathe.

I wasn't doing it alone and that truth steadied me more than any plan ever could.

In this moment, I acknowledge that sometimes having people around who understand your silence is all we need to pick ourselves back up again.

We must learn to focus on warm energy.
Soak our limbs in it.
Become better lovers of the world.

Because if we can't learn to be kind to the most desperate parts of ourselves, how will we ever truly understand the world? Most importantly when we stop trying to change everything and be present - what happens?

Vulnerability is the right choice
I've learnt all things come in twos:
Love & hate
Pain & Joy
Sugar & Salt
Life & Death.

So do me a favour - every morning you wake up, ask yourself:
What will make me feel loved, joyous , alive?

Not tomorrow.
Not next week.
But now.

12

Power of Showing Up

Success isn't about luck. It's a preparation meeting opportunity.

As someone who once studied Business and Management, that saying didn't sound smart - it was a wake up call.

I've learnt about risk registers, forecasting, contingency planning.

You always need a plan B, that will get you to your desired destination - no matter how many times you have to reroute.

Because no matter how solid your proposal was, life has its own ideas.

Sometimes things fall apart.

But the question is - do you sink or swim?

There are going to be days when you feel low.

When your energy is gone.

When you don't want to pick up the phone, go to the gym, leave your bed or show your face.

But you still have to show up.

Not for the world.

For you.

That's what success actually is.

It's not found in perfect conditions,

It's built in the uncomfortable moments were you show up anyway.

Showing up is how you earn your own trust.

There's an analogy I once shared:

Picture a window.

Every time you show up for yourself, you clean a small part of that glass.

The more consistent you are, the clearer your vision becomes.

But when you stop showing up, the window fogs.

Doubt settles in.

You stop seeing what's possible - because your view is blocked by inaction.

You can pray, plan and proclaim...

but none of it means anything if you don't move.

Because what is a goal without movement?

A dream without discipline?

A calling without consistency?

When I reflect on my journey, I realise:

It was about focusing on what was in my control.

It was about creating moments that prepared me for what I

couldn't yet see, in the ordinary moments.

I still face doubts.

I still adjust.

But I show up differently.

There's intention in my posture.

Purpose in my steps.

Not because the path is clear - but because I've decided to walk it anyway.

The world doesn't remember the ones who had potential.

It remembers the ones who showed up - again and again. Until it was undeniable.

13

Becoming at Home in My Body

It wasn't weight I needed to lose, it was disconnection.

As I practised gratitude and being present.

I also started to listen to my body in that stillness.

I had let myself go, not because I didn't care but I expected someone else to care before I did.

As I stared in the mirror one morning, I finally started to listen:

Just like that, an undeniable realisation arrived "I don't feel at home in my body anymore."

I wasn't chasing a number on the scale.

I wasn't compromising myself to anyone else.

I just felt… out of sync with myself.

Some morning I'd look in the mirror and think, this can't be it.

Not the shape.

The energy!

The tightness around my spirit, not just my clothes.

I missed feeling free inside my skin.

So I decided to change something.

Not everything.

Just something.

I started small.

A few squats.

Less sugar in my coffee.

A walk instead of scrolling.

I just wanted to prove to myself I still cared.

That I was still present in this body.

Still grateful for it even when I didn't always recognise it.

That's when I started reading Atomic Habits.

And what it taught me was this:

You don't need motivation. You need motion.

You don't need to overhaul your life. You need to cast a vote for the person you're becoming every single day.

So I did.

One healthy decision at a time.

One early morning gym session at a time.

One "you've got this" whisper at a time.

And little by little, I stopped fighting my body.

And started thanking it.

Feeding it without punishment.

Moving it without resentment.

The changes came slowly - then all at once.

Not just physically.

But emotionally.

I felt powerful.

Like I was finally walking in partnership with my body instead of apologising for it.

And I'll say this:

We live in a world that makes women feel like their bodies are public property.

Like you should edit it, slice it, filter it, hide it or flaunt it perfectly.

But what if you didn't?

What if you didn't rush to "fix" your body?

But instead sat with it long enough to understand it.

Here's what I know:

Sometimes it's not your body that needs to change.
It's your relationship with it.
This is not a chapter about weight loss.
This is a chapter about agency.
About choosing to love your body not just when it looks the way you want,
But when it's carrying grief, softness, hormones, motherhood, fatigue and survival.

III

The Becoming

Growth isn't always graceful. This was a stretch, the uncomfortable space where I had to face myself. Old patterns resurfaced. Resistance showed up. But so did clarity. In choosing alignment over approval and healing over habit, I began to shift my mindset and step into who I was always becoming, even when I didn't realise it.

14

Burn the Script

When you realise you're the one you've been waiting for.

I remember being back home with my parents. No real plan. No real idea of what was coming next.

Just me, a child, and a quiet storm in my chest that refused to go away.

On the outside, I was holding it together. On the inside, I was questioning everything - not from a place of defeat, but from a place of deep confrontation.

The truth is, I had lived far too long on autopilot.

Smiling when I wasn't okay.

Nodding through chaos.

Shrinking to survive.

I started noticing how many things I had normalised - dysfunction, emotional weight, even silence. And slowly I began waking up.

Not all at once. But thought by thought. Day by day.

I realised I had been tolerating things I had no business entertaining.

Living like life was just happening to me.

I was waiting for someone to rescue me when all along, it had to be me.

No one was coming.

And honestly, that truth hit hard - but it also set me free.

Becoming intentional wasn't some grand moment.

It was quiet and gritty.

It looked like choosing to show up when I wanted to disappear.

It sounded like asking myself questions I used to avoid.

It felt like peeling back layers and having no clue what I'd find - but going there anyway.

At some point, I got tired of my own patterns.

Tired of reliving the same lesson, just different people.

Tired of handing energy I hadn't even given myself.

I had to face it: the version of me I kept trying to protect was also the version holding me back.

So I stopped calling survival "strength."

I stopped begging for signs and started making decisions.

I started moving like I meant it - even when I was afraid.

Food for thought:

You see, it's easy to stay numb. But choosing to rise? That takes guts.

It takes believing in something you don't see and from a

psychological point of view - if you believe in God, there is no reason why you cannot believe in yourself.

Choose to lead even when you're scared. Because truthfully, no one's going to hand you your breakthrough. Even the Bible says, faith without the works is dead.

15

Check Your Attitude

The mindset that was quietly sabotaging me.

I didn't realise my attitude was the reason some things weren't moving.

Not my effort.

Not my ideas.

Not my ability.

My attitude!

That quiet voice said, "Why should I bother?"

The heavy sigh before starting something I claimed to care about.

The silent resentment I carried.

I used to think I was tired.

But deep down, I was ungrateful.

And ungratefulness has a smell.

It shows up in how you speak.

How you wait.

How you respond when things don't go your way.

It's easy to call yourself humble.
But the real test is how you act when things feel unfair.

Sometimes I'd secretly hope someone would notice me.
That someone would see I'm trying.
That they'd tell me I deserve better.

But that's not how elevation works.
It doesn't come with applause.
It comes with self-awareness.
And it starts with checking your attitude.

Ego will tell you "I know this already."
But wisdom says "There's always more to learn."

Pride will make you clap back.
Growth will make you pause.

And the truth?
A bad attitude can kill a good thing before it even begins.

Reflection:

Looking back, I realised I wasn't always ready - not because I lacked skill, but because my attitude wasn't in alignment with what I was asking for.
God had to humble me. Strip me. Quiet me.
And in that stillness, I finally saw the truth:

Elevation doesn't start with doing more.
It starts with becoming better.
I had to soften.
Let go of entitlement.
And choose character over performance.
Because where you're going, you can't carry a hardened heart.
Only a whole one.

16

Outgrowing Noise

Discernment doesn't always announce itself.

Lately, I've found myself quieter in rooms I used to pour into.
Not because I am angry.
Not because I think I am better.
But because I've changed.

Conversations I used to entertain no longer resonate.
Small talk feels smaller when you've tasted deep healing.
And surface level just doesn't sit the same after doing the inner work.

When I stopped being a yes-woman, the energy quietly shifted.
No dramatic exits.
No loud declarations.
Just... space.

I showed up with love - steady, grounded, clear.
But my confidence wasn't received the same.

People started stepping back, unsure of what to do with this new version of me.

The version that didn't neglect me.

Wasn't pleasing.

Wasn't waiting to be picked.

Saying "no" became a form of self-respect.

But to some, it felt like rejection.

And I had to make peace with that.

I realised some people preferred the broken version of me.

The one who overextended.

The one who proved her worth by showing up for everyone but herself.

The one who stayed in rooms longer than she should have, just to avoid discomfort of being misunderstood.

But that was never who I truly was.

That was the version I became to survive.

Now I honour my time.

I move with intention.

I love deeply - but no longer abandon myself in the process.

And no, silence isn't shade.

It's sacred.

Key takeaway:

Not every shift is a loss.

Some are sanctified re-directions, the kind only discernment can see and only peace can explain.

Growth doesn't come with closure.
Sometimes it arrives in silence, asking you to choose alignment over approval.
You don't need to explain your evolution to people committed to misunderstanding you.
You're not walking away - you're walking forward.
Real love won't require you to shrink.
And real peace?
It will never compete with noise.

17

The Child Within

We're all carrying something we never asked for.

Childhood trauma?

Some carry the heavy kind.
Others, the silent kind.
But the truth is - almost all of us carry it.

An unspoken wound.
A memory.
A moment where we felt unseen.
Unheard.
Unloved.

At some point in our childhood, something shifted.
Even if the people around us meant well.
Even if we had "enough."
The child within still remembers.

And then one day, you grow up.
You become an adult.
The friend.
The parent.
The guide.

And suddenly, you realise -
You can only give love in the way you received it...
Or in the way you had to teach yourself.

So what happens then?
Do you pass on what hurt you?
Or do you fight to break the chain?

Do you consciously repeat what once felt normal,
Or do you stand in the discomfort long enough to rewrite the pattern?

I look at my own daughter sometimes, and I know:
One day, I may disappoint her.
Not because I want to.
But because I am human.

No one was ever designed to be perfect.
Not you.
Not me.
Not them.

May you forgive those who hurt you - knowingly and unknowingly.
Not for them.

But to set yourself free.
Because love is the greatest expression of freedom.
Let it in.
Let it live through you.
Let it break the chain that was sent to destroy you.

Food for thought

The child in you deserved more.
But the adult in you gets to choose differently.
What have you been carrying that was never yours to hold - and are you ready to put it down?

A letter to my daughter

If there's ever a moment in your life when you feel like I've let you down - I want you to remember something.

I won't always get it right.

But I will always come back to love.

And every part of me that's trying to grow, is trying to do so because of you.

You're the reason I chose to break the cycle.

To love louder.

To listen better.

To feel everything I once ran from - just so you wouldn't have to.

I don't need to be perfect.

I just need to be present.

And I will always be that for you.

With all my heart,
Mom

18

The Run That Woke Me Up

Healing doesn't always look like rest. Sometimes, it looks like running toward the part of you that's been waiting to rise.

June 2024

I laced up my trainers and ran my first 5k for charity.

I didn't just cross a finish line - I crossed a threshold in my mind.

A quiet war I'd been fighting for years, finally felt like it had a face. And that day, I outran it.

I still remember the training.

The sweat.

The sore muscles.

The early mornings when it would've been easier to give in.

But something deeper kept going.

Each run wasn't just physical.

It was spiritual.

Therapeutic.

An unspoken prayer that only my body knew how to release.

While I trained, I fed my mind with motivational podcasts.
Not for hype but for mental toughness.
Because healing takes more than reflection.
It takes discipline.
Focus.
Commitment to the unseen.

With every gym visit, I felt lighter.
Not just in body but in spirit.
The frustration that once clung to me like a second skin started to melt away.

It felt like...
A clearing.
A reintroduction.
A becoming.

And in the middle of it all, one quote echoed louder than the rest:
"The tragedy of life is not death, but what we let die inside of us while we live" - *Norman Cousins*

That line became my anchor.
My silent whisper when doubt crept in.
When old thoughts tried to convince me to shrink.
When that voice said, "maybe you're not ready."
Or worse - "it's OK to quit while you're ahead."

But I've met failure before.

And I know what it isn't:
It isn't showing,
It isn't trying,
It's choosing to believe in yourself, even when you don't feel ready.

The truth is, if you're always waiting to be fully ready,
You'll never find out how life can surprise you.
Because serendipity can't meet you at the start line, if you never show up to run.

And when I crossed that line, I didn't just finish.
I remembered!

Affirmation for the one Becoming:
Don't do it to prove you're strong.
Do it because you're done negotiating with fear.

The resistance you feel isn't weakness - it's a threshold.
Push gently.
But push.

Discomfort isn't always a red flag.
Sometimes it's a signal that you've finally stopped avoiding yourself.

We need to be confident to start.
We need to be honest.
About what you've avoided.
And about what you're capable of even if you haven't seen it yet.

Growth rarely feels glamorous.

It feels like uncertainty, silence, shaky hands, and steady decisions.

You don't need applause.

You need consistency.

And one quiet moment of courage at a time.

This isn't about running.

It's about returning.

To your fire.

To your focus.

To the part of you that refuses to die quietly.

Try not because it's easy.

Try, because you deserve to see what happens if you don't give up this time.

To meet your best self, you must lose your weak self.

19

Old Habits Return

Not everything familiar deserves a second chance.

July 2024.

Just when I thought moving back with my parents was enough surrender.

She came back!

The version of me I used to wear like perfume.

Soft, familiar, dangerous.

A few weeks after that quiet revelation in July, a friend visited.

They suggested a night out.

And the old me - the one who still liked to flirt with fire - whispered,

"Say yes. What's the harm?"

The part of me still craved something outside of myself said,

"Come on... just for fun."

And I said yes.
As I got dressed,
I didn't just wear clothes -
I wrapped myself in unfinished healing.
The outfit looked good.
But it was hiding something fragile:
The inner girl who was still learning that confidence isn't found in mirrors.
It's forged in silence.
In alignment.
In truth.

I looked at myself and thought:
They'll say I'm glowing.
But what they couldn't see
was the part of me still aching.
Still unsure.

The music played.
The world spun in artificial light.

But inside me, something asked.
Are you healing or are you revealing your scars?

I smeared on foundation
Lipstick.
Flicked my hair just right.
And as I looked into the mirror,
there she was again -
the old me!

Ego rose like a shadow in stilettos and whispered,
"You only live once."
And maybe that's the most toxic sentence we feed ourselves.
To justify the slow erosion of a decision we know doesn't belong to us anymore.

It's not that going out is wrong.
There is a season for joy.
A season for dancing.
A season for play.

But this wasn't that season.

This season was solitude.
A quiet road that asked me to shed the things I once used to feel alive -
because I now knew were masks.
Temporary confidence boosters.
Emotional placeholders.

And I was finally ready to put them down.

This is what I now know:
As long as we seek worth from anything outside of us.
We hand the keys of our happiness
to people, places, and moments,
that were never built to carry it.
Confidence without alignment is performance.
Healing without honesty is delay.
And love without truth... is theatre.

20

When Love Looks You In The Mirror

It wasn't love I wanted, it was validation.

Not the idea of it. Not the version that flatters your ego. The real thing - starting with you.

After that night out,
I sat back down.
Not physically - spiritually.
And this time, I didn't run.

I asked myself the question that most of us avoid:
Are you ready to love yourself as you are?
I don't mean a 10 step facial routine.

At first, I told myself I just wanted to be loved.
But then I dug deeper.
Do you want to be loved or do you like the idea of it?
Because love - real love, asks for honesty.
It won't compete with fear.

And it can't survive the games you play to see if someone's going to prove you wrong.

If I really wanted love,
Why do I keep testing it?
Poking at it?
Doubting until it's broken.
Just to comfort myself with the lie that "I was right all along."

Right about what?
That love doesn't last?
That no one stays?
That I'll never be fully understood?

That's not true.
That's trauma.

And if it wasn't love I was chasing,
maybe it was just the idea of it.

Someone to fill the silence.
Someone to buy the flowers.
Someone to make life feel a little less boring.
Aesthetic affection - curated for the gram.
A fallback for empty Sundays and late-night doubt.

But here's what I had to ask myself:
Do I even give that to me?
Do I take myself out with intention?
Sit in beautiful places because I believe I deserve them?

Buy myself flowers, not to post,
but to honour my presence.

Do I whisper "I love you" to the mirror
with the same conviction I give to others?
Because how can I receive what I haven't even learned to offer myself?

That question didn't bring textbook answers.
It brought experience.
It brought unlearning.
It brought me face to face with a truth I had danced around for years.

Love starts with what you do in private.
How you talk to yourself when you feel unworthy.
What you believe about yourself when no one is watching.
What you tolerate -and what you refuse to carry forward.

And what unfolded after that question...
was more than I ever imagined.
Because when you stop running from yourself,
you stop chasing love that isn't rooted in truth.

What I now know:

If no one ever brought me flowers again,
I would still believe I am worthy and beautiful.

If no one ever told me they loved me,
I would comfortably say it to myself and mean it.

This wasn't about rejecting love,
It was about building a version of me that wouldn't need to chase or beg for it.

Real love doesn't come to complete you.
It comes to join you.

Only when you've come home to yourself first!

21

Wisdom Through Her Eyes

Her peace showed me mine still needed work.

January 25

The day my daughter taught me how to let go without losing myself.

I didn't know a small playground moment would stay with me this long -

but it's the day my daughter taught me something I'll never forget.

We were out, just the two of us. The day felt light -

one of those moments where everything seems fine on the surface.

She was playing with a group of children,

completely in her own world - smiling, bubbling,

just being her joyful little self.

Then it happened.

One of the children snatched the toy she was holding.

No warning. No explanation. Just took it from her hands like it didn't matter.

I watched it unfold from a few steps away.

Everything in me wanted to react.

My first instinct as a mother? Step in. Say something.

Correct the child.

But something told me to wait.

To watch.

And in that moment, I witnessed something that nearly brought tears to my eyes.

My daughter didn't scream.

She didn't cry.

She looked down, visibly sad for a moment -

maybe a minute or so.

You could see it had touched something in her.

But then - just like that, she looked around,

found another toy, and started playing again.

Happy.

Content.

Just as she was before.

I froze, but this time it wasn't because of shock.

It was pride.

It was a revelation.

I saw something so pure in her response -
something I hadn't even mastered in my adult years.
She didn't internalise loss.
She didn't retaliate or let it ruin her day.
She let go and moved on.
She chose joy again.

And I'll be honest - I don't know if I would've done the same.

The day taught me a hard, holy truth:
She's stronger than I sometimes giver her credit for.
And strength doesn't always look loud or defiant.
Sometimes, it looks like choosing joy anyway.

That's when I realised,
My job as her mother isn't to protect her from every moment like that.
It's to prepare her for them.

Because the world may take things from her.
Sometimes unfairly.
Sometimes without reason.
Sometimes right out of her hands.

And I won't always be there to stop it.

But if I can raise her in love,
nature her self-awareness,
and equip her with strong, rooted mindset.
She'll know how to bounce back every single time.

Her response was a mirror for me.
How many times in life had I held onto things too long?
How many times had I made pain my identity?
How many times did I stop playing - just because something had been taken from me?

But she reminded me:
You can feel loss and still choose joy.
You can acknowledge the moment and still carry on.

So no, it wasn't just a toy.
It was a turning point.
Not in her but in me.
Because I saw the fruit of something I had prayed to build in her:
resilience that doesn't require revenge.
Joy that doesn't beg for justice.
Peace that doesn't need to prove anything.

So if this has ever been you:
A reminder that you won that day.
Not because you got what you lost back but because you didn't let it take you with it.

You're light.
You're grounded.
You're already more powerful than you know.

And I pray you never lose that softness,
because that softness is your strength.

IV

The Return Home

This is where everything began to make sense, not because life got easier but because I finally remembered who I was. The journey inward led me to love, purpose and spiritual authority.
I no longer chased validation, I stood in legacy. This was the arrival: not a destination, but to myself.
Home was never a place. It was always within me.

22

The Strong One

Learning to be held without apologising for it.

If you have ever carried the title of "the strong, independent one," I know deep down that, you've suffered in silence more times than you can count.

Not because others are bad.

But because you mastered the art of carrying what breaks you while comforting everyone else.

You've listened to others cry while your own voice trembled behind the throat.

You've helped people solve problems while yours piled up quietly buried behind the smile, masked by the words, *"I'm fine."*

And when you finally whisper for help - when your knees buckle

just a little - what do they say?
"You're strong. You'll figure it out."

And you probably will.
But that doesn't mean you should have to.

There's a particular kind of ache that comes with being seen as capable but not as human.
It's subtle, but it's there.

That ache says:
"You're strong enough to hold everyone else… but not fragile enough to be held."
"You're the example… so you can't unravel."
"You're the one they will look up to… so don't look down."

But here's what I've come to realise:

Strength without softness becomes self-neglect.

And that kind of strength?
It doesn't serve God.
It replaces Him.

Let me be honest with you...

I recently put that title down. Not because I became weak but because I finally became free.

Free to say "Today, I don't want to lead. I want to lean."
Free to admit, "Yes, I can figure it out but right now I don't

have it all figured out and don't want to do it alone."

Free to show up in rooms without over explaining why I am not smiling the same way I did yesterday and overextending.

I no longer wear "strong" as a badge of honour.

Because sometimes…It's a cage.

A beautifully decorated one, but a cage nonetheless.

What I carry now instead is grace.

Grace to be unfinished.

Grace to ask for help.

Grace to collapse into God's arms when I don't have the answers.

I no longer seek applause for surviving.

I seek alignment with the truth that:

My strength is made perfect in weakness (2 Corinthians 12:9)

That verse is an anchor.

Paul didn't say "My strength is made perfect in perfection."

He said **weakness**.

Because that's where God shows off.

Final words of Wisdom for The Strong One:

Letting go doesn't make you less. It makes you real.

You don't always have to be the one holding the room together.

Sometimes, the room needs to hold you.

You are still powerful when you're on your knees.
You are still worthy when your voice shakes.
You are still valuable when you're not fixing things.

So today if you feel tired...
Put the cape down.
Take the crown off.
Let yourself rest.
Your softness is not your shame - it's your sanctuary.

And remember:
You are not just the strong one. You are the whole one.
Let them see you cry.
Let them see you breathe.
Let them see you be.
Because the real you?
She is more than enough - even when she's not strong.

23

Are You Over or Under-qualified?

When life becomes your greatest education.

I've often wondered why, so many of us feel under-qualified.

Because we don't hold a specific degree?

Because a piece of paper doesn't carry our name, stamped with approval from a system that was never designed with our journey in mind?

Let me ask you something…

Have you overcome heartbreak?

Disappointment?

Grief?

Betrayal?

Poverty?

Low self-worth?

Mental battles?

Single parenting?

Starting again with nothing?

Then you, my friend, hold a PHD in perseverance and that is not something any institution can teach.

We spend years believing we're not "there yet" - because someone somewhere convinced us that our experiences weren't good enough to be called wisdom.

But let's think about this logically for a moment.

You get hired for a job because you can solve a specific problem, right?

Well... the pain you've overcome?
The patterns you've broken?
The inner battles you've silenced?

That's real life knowledge.
That's lived intelligence.

And more than that - it's wisdom.

So if purpose is about service using your gifts to help others, then why are we so quick to dismiss the gift of our pain?

I used to think my purpose was to become something.
Now I know:
My purpose is to serve through what I've survived.

Because the very thing that broke you might be the key that unlocks someone else's healing.

And the joy you're fighting for now?
It may become the exact hope someone else needed in action.

"Blessed be the God... who comforts us in all our troubles, so that we may comfort those in any trouble with the comfort we ourselves receive from God."

- 2 Corinthians 1: 3-4

Your pain isn't wasted - it becomes someone else's pathway.

"You intended to harm me, but God intended it for good to accomplish what is now being done, the saving of many lives."

- Genesis 50:20

Joseph didn't need a title. His experiences were the preparation.

Final Thoughts + A Challenge:
If a PhD takes 5 years to acquire...
Then how many are you holding in your soul, just waiting to be recognised?

If every problem you've overcome points to a pattern...
Is that not your calling?

And if your purpose is to serve...
Are you still waiting for permission to do what you've already been equipped for?

Don't let the absence of credentials silence the presence of your calling.
God doesn't call the qualified -

He qualifies the called through fire.

So here's my final question:
What if the thing you've been disqualifying is the very thing God wants to use to set others free?

24

Surrender

The moment you truly let go, is the moment everything begins.

I've done the work.
I've reflected, healed, shifted and risen.
So you might wonder where am I now?

But here's what I need to tell you…
None of it mattered until I really surrendered.
Real surrender isn't passive.
It's not giving up - it's giving over.

It when I said:
" God, I don't know what I'm doing anymore. But I know You do.
And now I give it to you - because I no longer want to be the architecture of a life You've already designed."

I used to think surrender meant weakness.
That handing things over meant I'd lose control.

But here's the truth:

I was never in control.

I was managing - not mastering.

I was holding on tightly to things I was never meant to control.

Surrender was the moment I stopped, pretending I could handle it all.

And finally felt peace.

Here's what surrender actually sounds like:

"Lord, even if I don't understand, I'll still trust You."

"Even if it doesn't happen my way, let Your will be done."

"Even if I have to let go of what I thought I wanted, I know You never take without giving better."

That's not a weakness.

That's warfare in wisdom.

Because peace doesn't come when everything is perfect.

Peace comes when you let God be God - and stop playing both roles.

One of my favourite scriptures is;

"Trust in the Lord with all your heart and lean not on your understanding; in all your ways acknowledge Him, and He will direct your paths"

- Proverbs 3:5-6

Your understanding is too limited to build a limitless life.

"Be still and know that I am God."

- Psalms 46:10

Stillness is not stagnation.

It's divine confidence that God is working - even in your waiting.

A Prayer to Begin Now:

Father, I surrender not because I'm tired, but because I trust You.

I release the timelines, the pain, the questions, the pride, the fear, and every false identity I've clung to.

I no longer want to be in control, I want to be in alignment.

Let my plans bow to Your purpose. Let my striving turn into stillness. Let my confidence be built in You, not the world.

I am Yours. Move through me. Use me. Mold me.

In Jesus' name, Amen.

Moment for honesty:

What are you still holding that God is waiting for you release?

25

A Promise to Never Break

The legacy I carry, the woman I'm becoming, the vow I will not let go.

Letter to My Future Self

Hey, as we come to the end of this book - I want you to remember something.

This was the final goodbye to your old identity.
The version of you who shrank herself.
Who stayed silent to keep the peace.
Who carried others while wondering who would carry her.
Who tried to outrun her story instead of standing in.

You've already done the hardest part: you stopped pretending.

It's been uncomfortable, peeling back the layers, letting go of timelines, saying no, crying in silence, walking away from noise, and learning to sit in stillness.

But it was never wasted.

Because now... you're awake.

And this chapter?

You're not being carried by the waves anymore - you're centred in truth.

You're no longer learning about yourself - you know who you are.

You're no longer dimming your light - you're sharing it with the world.

Not to impress... but for impact and most importantly for the glory of God.

Because everything you've walked through - the grief, the battles, the healing, the isolation - it wasn't just for you.

It was for the woman still whispering "Is something wrong with me?"

It was for the mother who feels lost in the noise of everyone else's needs.

It was for the girl who never heard that she was enough.

Your life is proof that God uses ordinary people to carry extraordinary purpose.

And this book?

It's just the beginning.

I am declaring this as a bestseller - not for title but I know there are many others out there like me and God will bring us together through this testimony - 1 testimony shall become hundreds, thousands, to millions.

I see myself sitting across from a great interviewer, one day, who will make space for truth.

And beside me, my daughter - holding my hand.

Not watching me perform, but watching me walk in alignment.

Watching me honour God without needing to be perfect.

She'll find her own voice, her own truth.

But she will always know: "My mom walked first. And she never gave up."

I may not know exactly how the next chapter looks.

But I know who is writing it and it's no longer fear.

I walk forward now with fire in my chest and peace in my stride.

This was never just about healing.

This was about becoming the woman I was born to be.

26

Heart to Heart

From a Mother to a Mother

Dear Mom,

We never got to speak when your time arrived.

But if we had… I think I would've said:

I see you now.

Not just as my mother but as a woman.

A soul who carried things no one asked her to carry.

A heart that may have broken in places I'll never fully understand.

Growing up without you left a silence in me I didn't know how to name.

It created questions that echoed louder as I got older.

But now I'm a mother too…

I've felt the stretch and the sacrifice.

I understand something I couldn't before:
You can't give what you didn't receive.

And even love, when buried beneath survival, can feel like absence.
And still - I love you no matter what!

Not because I've erased the pain of not understanding certain things.
But because I've released the weight.

If you were here today, I'd sit beside you and hold your hand.
I wouldn't ask for an explanation - I'd offer understanding.
I'd tell you "You did what you could. And I honour that."

Because we're all just daughters trying to find our way back home - to ourselves, to love, to God.

I know your love didn't die.
It lives in me.
It lives in this book.
It lives in the way I hold my child.
In the gentleness I'm learning.
In the truth I'm no longer afraid to speak.

You planted a seed, even in absence.
And I'm the fruit - fully grown, finally whole.

Thank you for being the beginning of my story.
I'll carry both of us from here.

THE END!

27

THE END!

A note from Clarisa

I hope this book has inspired you to take action, to start your journey.

If you have started already, may this serve as a reminder that you're not alone.

Look forward to hearing all about your testimony! Feel free to reach out via social media using my full name.

"The moment you decide to show up for yourself is the moment everything begins to shift" - *Clarisa Washoma*

Appendix

Acknowledgments

To those who saw me, held me, and believed in the woman I couldn't yet see.

Writing this book has been more than storytelling.

It's been a sacred return.

To God.

To myself.

To everything I thought was lost, but was actually being redefined.

To God - my anchor, my healer, my Father.

You pursued me when I was drifting, whispered to me in silence, and waited patiently until I was ready to surrender. This book is nothing without You.

I no longer chase outcomes - I follow Your peace. And I trust that where You lead, purpose will meet me.

To my daughter - you are the heartbeat of this book.

Your presence called forth strength in me I didn't know I had. Every chapter I wrote, I imagined you one day reading these pages, not just to understand me but to understand yourself.

You've changed the way I speak, think, pray and love.

You are my greatest why.

To my mother - even in your absence, your story lives on.

You've shaped me more than you'll ever know.

This book closes a chapter of grief and opens one of legacy.

To every woman who's ever asked "Is Something Wrong with Me?

This was for you.

Your pain is not shame.

Your healing is not selfish.

Your voice matters.

Your softness is still strength.

And your story? It's still being written by the hand of a God who never stopped loving you.

To my family, friends, strangers turned sisters, and everyone who shared a moment, a message, or a tear with me.

Thank you for listening, for witnessing, for walking beside me even from a distance.

And to the version of me who wrote this book in quiet rooms, late nights, and broken moments - you kept going.

You didn't wait for perfection.

You just told the truth.

And that truth has set you free.

This is not the end.

This is only the beginning!

With every word,

Clarisa Washoma

Index of Sources & Inspiration

Clear, James

Atomic Habits - Referenced for guidance on identity, habit formation, and everyday transformation.

(See: Becoming at Home in My Body)

Cousins, Norman

Quote: The tragedy of life is not death, but what we let die inside of us while we live."

(See: The Run That Woke Me Up)

The Holy Bible (NIV)

Scriptures referenced for spiritual context and reflection:

- Psalms 119:105
- 2 Corinthians 1:3-4
- 2 Corinthians 12:9
- Psalm 46:10
- Proverbs 3:5-6
- Genesis 50:20
- John 13:7
- Romans 8:28
- Hebrews 11:1
- James 2:17

These scriptures shaped and sustained the journey behind this book. May they bring light to yours as well.

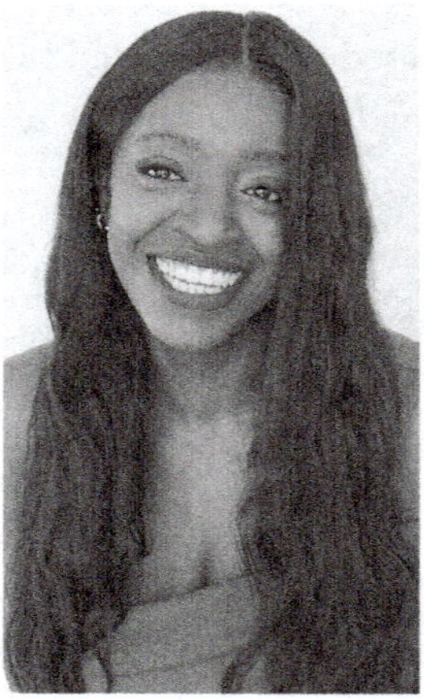

About the Author

Clarisa Washoma is a story teller, public speaker for positive mindset, and creative force whose journey from brokenness to breakthrough has inspired many to reclaim their power. Once burdened by self-doubt, emotional trauma, and the pressure to perform, she chose to confront her truth and start again but this time from inside out. What began as a personal search for identity and healing evolved into a life of purpose rooted in authenticity, courage, and faith. Through deep reflection, powerful mindset shifts, and unwavering self-belief, Clarisa transformed her pain into wisdom and her voice into a tool for change. *Is Something Wrong with Me?* is her raw, soul-stirring offering to the world, a blend of memoir and life guide for anyone ready to rise above their circumstances and walk boldly in who they were always meant to be.

You can connect with me on:

🔗 https://www.instagram.com/clarisawashoma?utm_source=ig_web_button_share_sheet&igsh=ZDNlZDc0MzIxNw==

Printed in Dunstable, United Kingdom

66860779R00067